Miraculous

CBD
The Essential Guide

Carol Merlo M.Ed.

Contents

Introduction

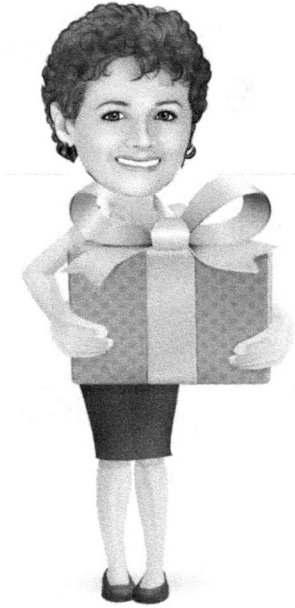

I am happy to welcome you to the next stage of your understanding of how you can impact your health using hemp CBD oils. This is a book about a remarkable substance that has been an intrinsic part of the human experience since the beginning of civilization. But with the ban on marijuana in the 1930's the benefits of hemp oil were suppressed until recently. These days, many of us know that CBD hemp oil is not the same as pot oil (which contains THC) and has a number of health benefits that people can receive without getting high.

I have been so impressed with this substance and how it worked for me that I have become a huge hemp advocate and want you to know only be informed but to spread the word about CBD oil and its benefits.

In case this is all new to you, the main difference between marijuana and hemp is the ratio of CBD to THC. The hemp plant has low levels of THC. Marijuana is specifically bred to have high THC content in the buds and flowers. In fact, the international definition of hemp is cannabis sativa that contains 0.3 percent or less THC. *(That's three tenths of one percent—virtually none!)*

So, enjoy the journey and let me know how CBD oil is working for you!

2

What Is CBD Hemp Oil?

Cannabidiol (CBD) oil is a natural, highly concentrated compound derived primarily from the seeds of the cannabis sativa plant. The hemp plant renders an oil that contains a combination of compounds that are unique to the plant, like CBD, with traces of THC, CBG (cannabigerol), CBCV (cannabidivarian), as well as compounds that exist in many other nutritious plants like amino acids, omega-3 oil, vitamins, chlorophyll, and terpenes—which are the compounds that evoke fragrance and have many healthful properties. This combination of compounds is what makes CBD hemp oil unique.

The benefits of CBD hemp oil have taken the health world by storm in recent years after being discovered in the 1990's. In study after study, CBD continues to prove itself as a potent agent for therapeutic use for conditions like cancer, diabetes, Crohn's disease, autoimmune diseases, rheumatoid arthritis, cardiovascular disease, chronic pain, PTSD, schizophrenia, multiple sclerosis, ADD, epilepsy, and more.

The United States first took notice of the research that was being conducted in the mid nineteen-nineties and issued a patent on cannabinoids in 1999, stating that *"Cannabinoids have been found to have **antioxidant properties**, unrelated to NMDA receptor antagonism. This new-found property makes cannabinoids useful in the treatment and prophylaxis of wide variety of oxidation associated diseases, such as ischemic, **age-related, inflammatory, and autoimmune diseases**. The cannabinoids are found to have particular application as **neuroprotectants**, for example in limiting neurological damage following ischemic insults, such as stroke and trauma, or in the **treatment of neurodegenerative diseases**, such as Alzheimer's disease, Parkinson's disease, and HIV dementia. Non-psychoactive cannabinoids, such as cannabidiol, are particularly advantageous to use because they avoid toxicity that is encountered with psychoactive cannabinoids at high doses useful in the method of the* *present invention."*

This led to a change in how CBD oil was viewed by the public and hemp oil is now widely considered to be a dietary supplement and manufacturers began to develop products that contain CBD and make them available for human and animal consumption. However, from a legal standpoint, the marketing of these products limits the use of the word CBD. Instead, you will find that a search on 'hemp oil' will render more results and those companies that are marketing these products are being careful not to cross the line that might lead to a perceived violation of Class 1 of the Controlled Substances Act, which is the categorization of cannabis that currently exists and includes CBD. Regardless, you can purchased CBD oil products legally in all 50 states without worry.

How CBD Works in the Body

The scientific discovery of the mechanism of hemp's incredible healing powers happened in 1990, when Dr. Raphael Mechoulam, a professor of medicine at the Hebrew University of Jerusalem in Israel (who just happened to also be the researcher who discovered THC), and his team were studying the brain. They found a special kind of neurotransmitter inside the brain they called anandamide, which is a *cannabinoid* that the body makes. Just as the body makes endogenous endorphins, it makes cannabinoids. And, just like opium is a phyto-endorphins, cannabis and some other plants make cannabinoids. The body makes its own cannabinoids and endorphins but cannabinoids are also found in plants like cannabis—hence the name.

The team went on to discover an entire network of cannabinoids and cannabinoid receptors throughout the human body, called the *Endocannabinoid System* or ECS. Thousands of studies now show that the endocannabinoid system is just as important as any other system, when it comes to human health. Cannabinoids and their receptors can be found in the brain, organs, glands, immune cells, and connective tissues. The primary purpose of this system is to maintain balance in the body, particularly with the hormones and neurotransmitters. To learn more about the Endocannabinoid System, read my book The Hemp Miracle.

CBD and Your Health

It is important to understand the role of nutrition in immune system health and hormonal balance when discussing the value of CBD. My book Create a Happy Body discussed the value of dietary supplements in maintaining long-term health. One of the most important dietary supplements you can take is Omega 3. Omega 3 fatty acids are required for the body to support cognitive and hormonal health, among other things. Omega 3s are also precursors to the production of endocannabinoids. In fact, without sufficient Omega 3, the CB1 receptors can break down. [1]

Unfortunately, with the lack of nutrient-dense food and the amount of toxins in our environment, the body cannot always make enough endocannabinoids and most of us are deficient.

This relationship between the need for phytocannabinoids and deficiency of endocannabinoids has been researched thoroughly and the term 'Clinical Endocannabinoid Deficiency Syndrome' has been coined to describe the manifestations of this lack and certain health conditions like migraine, fibromyalgia, and IBS, among others. [2]

So, I hope I have driven home the understanding that CBD oil is not just for people with health problems. It is important to nourish yourself with CBD so you can maintain your health and keep life-threatening conditions from rearing their ugly heads. Even though the body seeks out its own endocannabinoids, anyone who wants to maintain health and well-being should supplement with plant-based nutrients if they want to correct the imbalances of life's stresses, manage toxins, and offset dietary deficiencies. If we give our bodies the foods they need to support our systems, we can reduce and often eliminate chronic illness and medical bills. This includes a high quality fish oil supplement and CBD oil.

How CBD Benefits Specific Health Concerns

Anxiety

CBD has been shown to reduce anxiety in people with social anxiety disorder and it may also be effective for panic disorder, obsessive compulsive disorder, and post-traumatic stress disorder. *Social anxiety* is a medical term for people who are nervous in social situations. The greater social anxiety a person has, the more difficult it is for them to maintain eye contact or initiate and maintain a conversation. While everyone experiences situational shyness at some point, social anxiety disorder is a medical condition that can be attributed to about half of the people who have any social fears.

One of the ways to assess stress or fear in the body is to measure cortisol levels in the blood. Cortisol is one of the key hormones involved in inflammation and stress. Cortisol levels are heightened when animals are under extreme stress. A group of Brazilian researchers investigated the effect of CBD doses on human cortisol levels in humans and found that CBD decreased cortisol levels significantly more than a placebo.

One group of researchers studied the effects of a simulated public speaking test on healthy control people who took either CBD or a placebo 1.5 hours before making a speech. [3] These people had never been treated for social anxiety. The results showed that those people who took the CBD **improved their speech performance and significantly decreased their stress** when anticipating their speech. The placebo group showed greater anxiety, cognitive impairment, and discomfort. *They did MRI scans of the subjects afterward that revealed that CBD triggers activity in the areas of the brain that are linked to anxiety and*

7

emotion.

When you take CBD hemp oil, the cannabidiol (CBD) in it acts as an anxiolytic (anti-anxiety) agent by modulating certain neurotransmitters. Essentially, it inhibits 5-HT1A receptor sites which are found in high densities in the central nervous system and brain. CBD activates the receptors to trigger the release or inhibition of norepinephrine, which provides antidepressant, anxiolytic, and neuroprotective effects hence reducing anxiety. [4] Researchers conducting this research also discovered that 5-HT1A receptors were more involved in reducing anxiety compared to cannabinoid receptors such as CBl and CB2.

CBD oil inhibits anandamide deactivation, which improves both antipsychotic and anxiolytic (anti-anxiety) effects, and so can be useful in treating schizophrenia. It is important to note that only low to moderate doses, but not high doses, have been associated with anxiolytic effects. [5] Additionally, this oil reduces learned fear such as phobias and post-traumatic stress disorder; it does so by acutely reducing fear expression and disrupting reconsolidation of fear memory hence enhancing fear extinction.

Usage:

Ingest 3 drops of 2-5% CBD hemp oil in the morning or in the evening until all anxiety symptoms completely disappear.

Sleep

Have you noticed that when you have more stress, your quality of sleep is impaired? Sleeping well is fundamental to health and well-being.

People typically underestimate the health value of sleep. We know we need it to feel rested but sleep has an additional function that is critical to your health. During deep sleep, your body repairs itself. Your brain produces hormones and enzymes that you need to regulate every bodily system while you're sleeping. This is when the brain and the immune system does its work, so if you're awake and not sleeping well, you're missing out on the opportunity for your body to help regulate your health.

Studies of blood tests have shown that CBD oil impacts the dopamine levels in the bloodstream during sleep. This leads to a better, more relaxed sleep. Several studies have shown that CBD can have an effect on insomnia.

CBD doesn't just makes falling asleep easier, it also influences the sleep cycle. Sleep is divided into multiple cycles with different phases. CBD oil increases the third phase, which is that of deep sleep. In addition, CBD decreases the duration of REM sleep, which is a phase of light sleep during which dreaming occurs. REM sleep is necessary but too much of it causes fitful, light sleep. By reducing REM sleep, people dream less, memory is improved, and symptoms of depression are reduced.

In a 1981 Brazilian study, researchers assigned 15 insomniacs to a CBD dose (ranging between 40 mg and 160 mg), a placebo, or a drug used to relieve anxiety and insomnia. [6] With the highest CBD dose, sleep significantly increased, although dream recall was reduced, when compared to the placebo, indicating a deeper sleep.

Pain and Inflammation

According to the New England Journal of Medicine, more than 30% of Americans have some form of either acute or chronic pain and over 40% of older adults in the US have chronic pain. [7] There are three classes of drugs that work to reduce pain: over the counter analgesics like aspirin and NSAIDS, corticosteroids, and opiates.

The numbers are staggering. Sales in the US alone for OTC analgesics in 2016 was over four billion dollars! An estimated 9 million epidural steroid injections are performed annually in the US to relieve back and joint pain. Opiate use has become pandemic, often triggered by pain medication that is prescribed after an accident or surgery. Opioid analgesics are now the most commonly prescribed class of medications in the United States. In 2014 alone, U.S. retail pharmacies dispensed 245 million prescriptions for opioid pain relievers.

In our attempts to manage pain through the use of drugs, our population is experiencing adverse side effects leading to death and increased levels of addiction. This, if nothing else, is one of the most important reasons why people need to become educated about hemp and CBD.

When it comes to anti-inflammatory effects, CBD is a clear winner over drugs. A *proinflammatory cytokine* is a type of signaling molecule that is excreted from immune cells and certain other cell types that promote inflammation. A 2006 study showed a significant reduction of blood levels of *pro*-inflammatory cytokines when using CBD. So, **CBD reduces the levels of inflammation in the body**. Externally, it can be used as a topical ointment that relieves nerve pain and tingling in hands and feet.

Studies even suggest that CBD oil can reduce arthritis pain. A 2012 study published in the Journal of Experimental Medicine found that CBD significantly suppressed chronic inflammatory and neuropathic pain in rodents without causing analgesic tolerance. In other words, **you don't need**

to continue to increase the dose to get a response. [8]

CBD has also shown that it connects to the same brain synapses as opioids. This is big news, because **when used in conjunction with an opiate, CBD will reduce the likelihood of opiate dependence.** Whether your chronic pain is from an initial injury (like back sprain), brain cells responsible for stopping pain not working, or by an unknown cause, CBD oil can help address the pain.

Usage

Ingest 2.5-20 mg of CBD hemp oil, 2 times a day. Start will low amounts (say 5 mg) and then double it after every week.

CBD and the Heart

Heart disease is the leading cause of death in the US, with cancer as a close second. So, if CBD can protect the cardiovascular system the way it helps with pain, we have another miracle from hemp. A review of the literature in the British Journal of Clinical Pharmacology suggests a number of benefits to the cardiovascular system when taking CBD.[9] First, "CBD has direct actions on isolated arteries, causing both acute and time-dependent vasorelaxation." *Vasorelaxation* is the expansion of blood vessels so that more blood can flow at a lower pressure. Restricted blood vessels contribute to problems in heart disease. Researchers found that **CBD relaxes blood vessels so blood can flow more easily.**

CBD also **protects against heart tissue damage** caused when the blood supply returns to the tissue after a period of *ischemia*—which is *a* lack of oxygen—and against *cardiomyopathy*, like an enlarged heart or other heart tissue damage associated with diabetes.

Finally, CBD **protects against the blood vessel damage** caused by a high glucose environment, inflammation, or the induction of type 2 diabetes in animal models. One of the most common examples of this benefit is in diabetes, where vision and circulation problems cause pain and damage.

Diabetes

According to the *Centers for Disease Control*, almost ten percent of the people in the US are diabetic and another third of Americans are *pre-diabetic*. This is a phenomenal number of people whose health is adversely impacted by their diet and lifestyle and, as the population grows, this will only become a larger issue. But there is hope. For example, a 2006 study found that CBD treatment significantly reduced the incidence of diabetes in non-obese diabetic mice from an incidence of 86 percent in non-treated mice to an incidence of 30 percent in CBD-treated mice. [10] Researchers from the Hadassah University Hospital of Jerusalem examined the effects of CBD on development of diabetes in non-obese mice. For 26 weeks, they treated the mice with 10 to 20 injections of CBD oil (5 mg per kg body weight). The researchers discovered that compared to the untreated mice, the treated mice had reduced symptoms of diabetes. They suggested that CBD oil could treat diabetes because of its immune modulating effects that help prevent autoimmune diseases such as diabetes. CBD also increases the circulating endocannabinoids in the body, leading to improved endothelium dependent vasorelaxation, a condition that prevents diabetes.

That news is very helpful for people with diabetes but what about people who are pre-diabetic? In 2013, the American Journal of Medicine published a study that highlighted the impact of marijuana use on glucose, insulin, and insulin resistance among U.S. adults. [11] The study included 4,657 adult men and women from the *National Health and Nutritional Examination Survey* from 2005 to 2010. 579 of the subjects were current marijuana users and 1,975 were past users. The researchers found that current marijuana use was associated with 16 percent lower fasting insulin levels. They also found significant associations between marijuana use and smaller waist circumferences.

Chronic inflammation plays a key role in the development of insulin resistance, which leads to type 2 diabetes. Consequently, because CBD reduces inflammation it could also help improve the body's metabolism.

Usage

To help treat any type of diabetes and protect yourself from all the harm this disease can cause on your body (for example, insulin resistance, kidney damage, macro-vascular complications), take 25-30 mg of CBD oil every day.

Cancer

We all have cancer cells in our bodies at any time. These cells proliferate depending upon the health of our immune systems. The way the body eliminates them is through a process called *apoptosis*, which is essentially damaged cell suicide. If the process of apoptosis fails, the mutated cells can duplicate rapidly, invading the adjacent cells, which is what we call cancer. When our immune systems are healthy, they can recognize damaged cells and trigger apoptosis. One of the most exciting areas of research on CBD is its effect on cancer.

There are lots of studies on CBD and how it protects the body against cancer. In one study, investigators found that CBD protected DNA from oxidative damage and increased endocannabinoid levels. The National Cancer Institute details several studies into the anti-tumor effects of CBD. One study in mice and rats suggest CBD *"may have a protective effect against the development of certain types of tumors."* It may do this by inducing apoptosis, inhibiting cancer cell growth, and by controlling and inhibiting the spread of cancer cells.

Another study done by California Pacific Medical Center suggests that CBD "turns off" the gene involved in the spread of breast cancer. [12] They also found that CBD targets breast tumor cells and leaves healthy cells alone. Breast cancer experiments show that the number of cancer cells diminishes as more CBD is used.

CBD has been shown to be non-toxic in doses as high as 700 milligrams per day for 6 weeks, which means that it can be used for prolonged treatment and has potential for being developed into a drug for the treatment of cancer.

Not only does the research show that CBD is effective in fighting breast cancer cells, it also suggests that **it can be used to inhibit the invasion of cancer cells in the lung and colon.** Plus, it has demonstrated **anti-tumor properties in brain tumor studies as well as prostate, liver, pancreatic**

tumors, and even leukemia, where it has been proven that cannabinoids inhibit the growth of cancer cells.

Another important issue when it comes to the treatment of cancer, is its effect on the reaction to chemotherapy. **CBD eases nausea and vomiting.** Researchers have found that in low doses, it suppresses toxin-induced vomiting, but in high doses it increases nausea or has no effect. So, low doses of CBD are enough to ease the nausea from chemotherapy.

Although researchers are yet to agree on the effects of CBD on human cancer patients, many studies done on animals have proven that both THC and CBD possess anti-cancer properties. For example, a 2006 study done in Italy saw researchers inject human breast cancer cells onto the skin of mice to test the potency of the cannabinoids in hemp plant in inhibiting the growth of breast cancer.[13] The researchers discovered that CBD was the most potent cannabinoid.

The same researchers did another study where they injected human breast cancer cells into the paws of animals to test the relationship between CBD and lung metastases. They found that CBD had antitumor effects caused by apoptosis induction.

Usage
To treat skin cancer, start with 4-5 grams of this oil and double the amount after every week until you get to 30 grams. Apply the CBD oil onto your skin, cover it with a new, clean bandage after every 3 to 4 days.

For other types of cancer, ingest 60 mg of CBD oil (for starters) and continue increasing the amount until you get to 180 mg for 5 to 6 months. Note that some forms of cancer respond favorably to a combination of THC and CBD.

Epilepsy

Epilepsy is a condition that has shown a particularly beneficial response to CBD. A 2014 survey conducted at Stanford University was given to parents belonging to a *Facebook* group dedicated to sharing information about the use of cannabidiol-enriched cannabis to treat their child's seizures. [14] There was an average of 12 anti-epileptic drugs tried before using CBD. 84 percent of the parents reported a reduction in their child's seizure frequency while taking CBD. Of these, two reported complete seizure freedom, eight reported a greater than 80 percent reduction in seizure frequency, and six reported a 25–60 percent seizure reduction.

Later in 2014, researchers reported on preliminary results of a study involving children with treatment-resistant epilepsies. [15] People received a purified 98 percent CBD oil extract. After 3 months of treatment, 39 percent of the subjects had a greater than a 50 percent reduction in their seizures.

These preliminary results support the animal studies and survey reports that CBD may be a promising solution for treatment-resistant epilepsy.

Usage

Take up to 25 milligrams per kilogram of body weight. That is—if you weigh 100 pounds, you can take 1,136 mg of CBD per day and do just fine.

Schizophrenia

Psychosis is a loss of contact with reality. Step psychosis back and you have neurosis, which is depression, anxiety, obsessive behavior, or hypochondria, but without the radical loss of touch with reality. Research in this area shows that CBD has a pharmacological profile like that of certain antipsychotic drugs. People with psychotic episodes regularly show signs of endocannabinoid deficiency. They have fewer CB2 cannabinoid receptors than do healthy people. They also have lower levels of the enzymes that enable the endocannabinoid system to function properly. In 2012, the first controlled study on CBD and schizophrenia was done at the University of Cologne where 42 patients suffering from acute schizophrenia participated in the study. [16] Twenty one of them received 800 mg of CBD (orally) for 4 weeks and the other 21 received a standard medicinal drug amisulpride (a potent antipsychotic) for the same duration. Both treatments led to significant clinical improvement but the patients who received CBD treatment had increased blood anandamide levels.

Usage

Take 40-1, 280 mg of CBD oil by mouth 2 times a day.

Acne

A 2014 study published by the National Institutes of Health [17] stated that CBD hemp oil has a beneficial effect on acne. This is possible because CBD oil has antiseptic, anti-inflammatory, and sebum reducing properties that work together to reduce acne.

CBD oil increases cannabinoids such as (N-Arachidonoylethanolamine), which reduces the production of sebum. When sebum is produced in excess, it blocks skin pores and causes acne.

Further, the terpenes in CBD oil (such as limonene, linalool, and pinene) have antibacterial properties that act on the skin to reduce and prevent other acne effects such as pimples, redness, and pain.

Usage

Apply CBD hemp oil on the infected skin area 2 times a day.

Glaucoma

Glaucoma is an eye condition that causes intraocular pressure in the eye and that at the onset, has no noticeable symptoms. When left untreated, patients start experiencing symptoms such as nausea, vomiting, and pain. The increase in pressure can damage optic nerve, leading to loss of eye-sight.

A study done in 2004 showed that CBD oil **effectively lowers the intraocular pressure (IOP) and has neuroprotective actions, so is good for glaucoma.** [18] According to a pilot study done on 6 patients who had high intraocular pressure and ocular hypertension, half received a sublingual dose of CBD oil while the other half received a placebo.

After 2 hours, compared to those who had received placebo, the patients given CBD oil had lower intraocular pressure. The researchers concluded that CBD oil reduces intraocular pressure. It also reduces symptoms associated with glaucoma thanks to its anti-inflammatory properties.

Usage
20-40 mg of CBD oil sublingually, 2 times a day.

You can also put 1 or 2 drops l directly into your eyes every morning and evening.

Do not take more than 40 mg. to avoid an increase in pressure.

How Much Should I Take?

While I have provided amounts that have worked in studies for various conditions, the fact remains that everyone is different so what works for one person may not work for you. The serving size or amount of CBD will differ for each person, and even vary for the person depending on the state of their health and stress levels that day. Everyone reacts differently to various supplements, too.

Remember that CBD oil products are, by FDA guidelines, *food supplements.* As such, all products are required to have some form of nutritional label on them just like you'd see on food at your grocery store. And, all nutritional labels require a "suggested serving size." But just because this is requirement, it doesn't mean you have to follow those directions to the tee. You are in charge of noticing how varying amounts work for you and working with it to get the right amount of 'food' into your body.

The same product name made by a different company may result in different effects. The mix of terpenes and the variety of plant may impact how you experience it. Different companies use different extraction processes and delivery systems, so one mg. from one product may be three mg. of another, depending on how bioavailable it is. So, bottom line...experiment and see what works for you.

I suggest that you start small and gradually increase your serving size until you experience the desired result. The first things to consider when determining your needs, are your weight and the severity of your condition. The bigger you are, the more CBD you'll typically have to take. And, the more severe the situation, the more CBD you'll have to take.

Try it this way, and see if that works for you:

1. Take 1 serving/dropper full of your daily amount in the morning and 1 serving in the evening.

2. Take it twice per day for the first 3-4 days to build

it up in your system.

3. After these first few days, drop back to once per day and see how you feel.

From this point forward, experiment until you feel good. If you do not experience a reduction of the symptoms after 3-4 weeks, you should increase the amount until you experience the desired result. You can also increase the number of times throughout the day you take it.

Are there any downsides to taking CBD?

While most people will not experience any problems using CBD oil, it can inhibit drug metabolism and the activity of some liver enzymes, such as cytochrome P450. So, if you are using pharmaceuticals please check with an open minded doctor before you decided to mix the two.

Usage Chart

Please use this guide as a general recommendation. Each person is different in their response.

Issue	Amount
Anxiety	5 mg, 3 times per day
Sleep	40-160 mg before bed
Chronic Pain	2.5-20 mg per day
Diabetes and Pre-Diabetes	25-30 mg per day
Skin Cancer	4-5 grams to start and double the amount every week up to 30 grams. Apply the CBD oil onto your skin, cover it with a new, clean bandage after every 3 to 4 days.
Cancer	60 mg of CBD oil (for starters) and continue increasing the amount until you get to 180 mg for 5 to 6 months.
Epilepsy	200-300 mg of CBD by mouth daily for up to 4.5 months
Psychosis	Take 40-1,280 mg
Acne	Apply to the infected skin area 2 times a day.
Glaucoma	20-40 mg of CBD oil sublingually, 2 times a day. Do not take more than 40 mg. or it will increase eye pressure.

The Forms of CBD and How They are Used

There are many ways to ingest CBD oil. CBD is commonly taken orally in a concentrated paste or drops/tincture formula that you put under your tongue. Other oral methods include capsules, mouth strips, chewing gum, sprays, and edibles such as chocolate bars. Many people also use CBD on their skin via lotions, balms, creams, or patches. What matters most is trying a few different approaches and seeing what works.

When you use CBD oil, the type, or even the number of receptors it will activate depends on how much CBD is in the oil, how it is ingested, what other compounds are in the oil, and how bioavailable that oil is.

Tinctures

Hemp CBD oil tinctures are made in various strengths and are created by diluting pure CBD into either and oil or alcohol. Depending on the product, it is sprayed, squirted, or dropped under the tongue and held in place for about 30 seconds before it is swallowed. Often these products are flavored to make them more enjoyable to consume. There is an entire range of products out there, in terms of quality. Be sure to do your homework and read this guide thoroughly before purchasing. Sublingual ingestion is the second fastest application method behind inhalation.

Because people are different, the time it takes for CBD oil to start working will vary from one person to the other. Don't be afraid to experiment. I can tell when I am getting enough when I don't have a 'whoosh' experience about five minutes after I use it. To me, that indicates that I am deficient at that time. You may have a different experience or none at all when you take it. But pay attention to your aches and pains to figure out how much to take.

Edibles

Edibles are a great way to get CBD into your body and it works great for children, who might not like it in the other forms. While it is virtually impossible to measure how much you are getting into your system this way, consider that as a dietary supplement which provides so many health benefits, you will feel better overall when eating CBD. There are some wonderful products on the market. You can get it in chocolate or jelly, in the form of gummy bears, or even infused in chewing gum. Because CBD that is added to food is often pure CBD without the terpenes (so it tastes better) and because the delivery system has typically not been altered from its original form, it will take longer (about 20-60 minutes) to produce the desired results. This also depends on how long it has been since your last meal and the amount of food you ate. If you are looking for the fastest results from this method of application, eat your CBD oil edibles on an empty stomach.

Capsules

CBD oil in handy and easy to swallow pills vary in quality and bioavailability. different milligrams of CBD. Like hemp CBD oil tinctures, CBD oil capsules come in various types and can be combined with other herbs and vitamins to enhance their benefits.

CBD-infused capsules take longer to take effect than sublinguals because it they are released into bloodstream in the intestines, and so it takes a while before you experience an effect. You must be sure that the delivery system is taken into consideration if you are using a capsule because it will affect how well you absorb it. For example, water soluble is usually better than fat soluble. You will experience something more quickly with a sublingual.

Topicals

CBD topicals absorb slowly and uniformly through the

skin and give you long lasting effects. If you are looking for effects that last longer, go for this application method. These are commonly used for peripheral aches and pains in the joints or in skin conditions like psoriasis or shingles. Topicals work on the skin and top layers of muscle, so will not work like something you ingest.

The topical application of cannabinoids allows them to be absorbed directly for localized relief of pain, soreness, and inflammation. The skin quickly absorbs lipid-based materials that make contact with it and therefore, this is one of the most effective ways to use cannabinoids. Salves and balms are usually stronger than lotions or creams and all topicals should be rubbed in thoroughly. If your product contains THC, it will not make you high.

When you apply the oil on your skin or hair, beneficial CBD oil properties such as vitamins, chlorophyll, omega fatty acids, and terpenes permeate into the body, leading to a smooth and radiant skin. Topical CBD oil is in form of moisturizers, cleansers, lotions, and salves.

Inhaling

CBD can be purchased and used in an e-cigarette or vaporizer in the same way that tobacco or cannabis is vaporized. Vaporizing CBD has a fast onset time so you can determine how much to take more easily. However, the effect does not last as long, so you will need to use it throughout the day. Vaporizing methods are usually not as strong as the straight oils, tinctures, or capsules, and so most people vaporize as an adjunct to their other CBD products.

What to Look for When Buying CBD

Before you make a financial commitment to a CBD product, make sure you are getting the best product for the money. Here are some things to look for when deciding if the product you are buying is going to deliver what it says it will: safety, standardization, extraction, and the delivery system.

When it comes to CBD oil, quality depends on the percentage concentration of cannabidiol and the delivery system in the oil. Price depends on a number of things like how it was grown, how it was extracted, and how the delivery system was produced. The higher the quality, the more powerful the results will be. You may be tempted to buy the most affordable CBD oil in the stores or online but always remember that 'cheap is expensive.' It is better to spend those extra dollars and get the best oil than to settle on cheap oil that will offer you zero benefits. I have had a number of people come to me saying that CBD oil didn't work for them. I immediately ask them how they decided on what they took because there are many options out there and you have to take a minute to find out if what you are taking is going to work or not.

Is it Safe?

Many products on the market can contain pesticides, herbicides, and mold. So be sure to check the product for the following:

Organic soil – It goes without saying that the quality of the soil determines the quality of the CBD or other food products. Hemp takes up toxins in the soil and water, so the growing conditions need to be controlled to prevent these toxins from showing up in the product. Even though hemp requires little to no pesticides, the soil on which it is grown may have residual toxins and heavy metals from the past or from the water being used for irrigation.

Is it Standardized?

If you grind up a plant—or in this case plant oil—and you put it in a pill or potion, what do you get? That depends on where it was grown, when it was grown, what the soil and water was like, and how it was processed. To make a high-quality product with a good shelf life, you need to ensure that each dose is consistent from batch to batch. That is called standardization. There are a couple of ways that a consumer can be assured that the product they are taking is standardized. The first way is to know that the company providing the product has a state-of-the-art laboratory where the product is tested for consistency. Transparency, in terms of the manufacturing process is critical to providing the consumer with standardization assurance. The second way is for the company to provide quality assurance data from a 3rd party lab and other certified sources.

Testing

GMP stands for Good Manufacturing Practices. In the US, the FDA specifies that GMP for dietary supplements means that the dietary supplement consistently meets the established specifications for identity, purity, strength, composition, and limits on contaminants, and has been manufactured, packaged, labeled, and held under conditions to prevent adulteration. Check for GMP certification. Good companies will test their product using equipment that measures toxin levels and consistent amounts of active component.

You should not trust any seller who is not willing to certify lab analysis for their CBD oil. If a seller is not willing to offer this certification, it means such a seller is trying to hide some information since this is the only way you can determine the purity, concentration, and psychoactive effects of the oil. Always look for a seller who is willing to answer all your questions about their CBD oil and only purchase when you are satisfied.

What has Been Added to the Oil?

100% CBD is extremely expensive and not normally needed so most manufacturers provide CBD in combination with other ingredients. For example, many manufacturers will add MCT oil. MCT stands for medium chain triglycerides which can come from either palm or coconut oil. Recent research has found that MCT oil is easy to digest and benefits cognitive function. [19]

CBD is also added into different dietary supplements that may have herbs or vitamins to enhance the properties of the supplement.

What has Been Removed from the Oil and How was it Extracted?

In an effort to provide efficacious CBD, companies have tried different methods for ending up with a standardized amount of product per dose. To get the most bioavailable and standardized amount of CBD in a product, the extraction process must be considered. There are many ways to extract CBD from the hemp plant. Some methods are safer and more effective than others. Some are less expensive than others.

Some processing methods destroy the terpenes and phytochemicals that work synergistically with CBD. However, some edibles and tinctures remove the terpenes and chlorophyll to improve the flavor profile. Terpenes are the fragrant oils that give plants their various aromas. In cannabis, the terpenes are mostly secreted in the flower's resin glands. Terpenes exist in hemp as well as in marijuana. Cannabis has about 140 different terpenes. Terpenes bind to receptors in your brain to give you various effects, just like cannabinoids do. Studies on terpenes from cannabis show that they are as responsible for the benefits to the body as is cannabidiol. For example, *e-myrcene*, the most abundant terpene in cannabis, has *analgesic* (relieves pain), anti-inflammatory, antibiotic, and *antimutagenic* (prevents cells from mutating) properties. Other terpenes act in a similar way that antidepressants do to mediate the function of the neurotransmitters *serotonin* and *norepinephrine*. They also increase *dopamine* activity, which helps people with focus, productivity, and motivation. Research has shown that ingesting pure CBD crystals does not render the same benefits as whole plant CBD oil, which has been minimally processed.

With that in mind, let's look at the primary ways that processors extract CBD from the plant:

co2 Extraction

The co2 method uses carbon dioxide under high pressure and extremely low temperatures to isolate, preserve, and maintain the purity of the oil and the terpenes. However, the equipment is expensive, so you might have to pay a bit more for CBD oil processed this way. Depending on the way it is processed, it may or may not retain the chlorophyll, which some people regard as having it taste bad. Given that co2 is a naturally-occurring pure chemical substance, it leaves behind no residue.

Ethanol (Solvent-based) Extraction

This process uses chemicals solvents like butane, hexane, alcohol, or other ethanol to extract the CBD from the hemp plant. This is a less expensive process than co2 extraction but the resulting product may leave behind a residue which can be harmful to people whose immune systems are already compromised. High grade grain alcohol can be used to create high quality cannabis oil. But this extraction method destroys the plant waxes, which may or may not have health benefits. It is also flammable.

Bioavailability

There are numerous companies on the market these days that promote their CBD products using confusing marketing language. So, here is my word to the wise: *Just because a company or promotional literature says it, it doesn't mean it's true!* There are many companies in the dietary supplement space that do not have what the bottle says they have. You will spend your hard-earned money on something that will not get you the benefits you are looking for unless you do your homework. So, if you want to get the biggest benefit from your buck, take a minute to be sure you know what you are getting.

A delivery system is the way in which a substance is made *bioavailable.* Bioavailability is the extent to which a substance is taken up by a specific tissue or organ after it is administered. Think about making a salad dressing. You typically mix an oil (fat) with an acid, like vinegar or lemon, and some herbs. But you have to shake the bottle to get any of the flavor; otherwise you are getting straight oil. If you want to get the oil and vinegar to mix together without having to shake them, you need an *emulsifier,* which binds the oil and vinegar together. For example, you can add mustard to emulsify your salad dressing.

Similarly, cannabinoids bind to fat, which makes them poorly soluble in water, and you need to take a higher amount to get the benefits you want. Blood consists mainly of water, so processors want to make sure that their cannabinoids are soluble in water and, therefore, also in blood. Otherwise, you have big fat globules floating around in your blood, not doing much benefit. So, it makes sense that when CBD is engineered to be water soluble, the amount of it that can be delivered into the cells is increased. And, when bioavailability is increased, more CBD makes it through the metabolic process so you need a smaller serving size to get the same result. So, to improve absorption and deliver a standardized amount of CBD oil, companies have come up with various unique methods for delivering standardized doses using either liposomes, hydrosomes, or micelles.

Liposomes

Liposomes are the result of the natural encapsulation of lipophilic (fat loving, like CBD) and hydrophilic (water loving, like blood). They are a very effective method of bypassing the destructive elements of the gastric system and aiding the encapsulated nutrient to be delivered to the cells and tissues and thereby increasing the bioavailability of the CBD oil.

Many nutrients have poor oral bioavailability. So, encapsulating these substances in liposomes is a very effective method for aiding in the delivery of the nutrients to the cells and tissues. Over 50 years ago, researchers discovered that they could fill liposomes with drugs to protect and deliver them into the body and even into specific cells of the body, so this technology is not new, but it is new to the dietary supplement industry.

Hydrosomes

Hydrosomes are tiny micro-clusters of water that are about roughly 1/10th the size of normal water clusters. When you swallow them, micro-clusters of water are easily absorbed into the blood and the cells. The logic behind hydrosomes is that liposomes vary in size and so could be slow to be absorbed into the body, depending on the method of ingestion. So, if you use a hydrosome, instead, you can determine the size of the particle that is to be absorbed and ensure the delivery of the particle.

Micelles

Micelles are **nano-sized clusters that improve the surface area for absorption of a substance. In this way, it can** reduce the surface tension between two liquids and act as an emulsifier, so this is perfect for oil based substances like CBD.

Conclusion

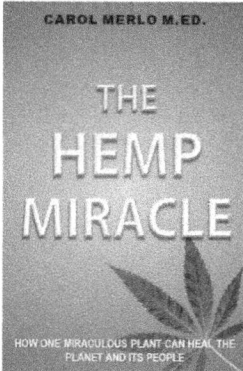

Thank you again for downloading Miraculous CBD! This book has highlighted all the amazing things that CBD oil can do for you. Take a deeper dive into the world of hemp. Discover its fascinating history and the numerous uses of the plants. Go online and get a 10% discount off the price of my book The Hemp Miracle at www.TheHempMiracle.com.

I appreciate all reviews on Amazon. This helps spread the word about the book and the value of this miraculous plant.

Thank you and good health!

Carol Merlo M.Ed.

References

1. Cannabinoid receptor-dependent and -independent anti-proliferative effects of omega-3 ethanolamides in androgen receptor-positive and -negative prostate cancer cell lines. Iain Brown, Maria G. Cascio, Klaus W.J. Wahle, Reem Smoum, Raphael Mechoulam, Ruth A. Ross, Roger G. Pertwee, and Steven D. Heys. Carcinogenesis. 2010 Sep; 31(9): 1584–1591.

2. Clinical endocannabinoid deficiency (CECD) revisited: can this concept explain the therapeutic benefits of cannabis in migraine, fibromyalgia, irritable bowel syndrome and other treatment-resistant conditions? Smith SC, Wagner MS. Neuro Endocrinol Lett. 2014;35(3):198-201.

3. *Cannabidiol Reduces the Anxiety Induced by Simulated Public Speaking in Treatment-Naïve Social Phobia Patients.* Bergamaschi MM, Queiroz RH, Chagas MH, de Oliveira DC, De Martinis BS, Kapczinski F, Quevedo J, Roesler R, Schröder N, Nardi AE, Martín-Santos R, Hallak JE, Zuardi AW, Crippa JA. Neuropsychopharmacology (2011) 36, 1219–1226; doi:10.1038/npp.2011.6;

4. *Agonistic Properties of Cannabidiol at 5-HT1a Receptors.* Ethan B. Russo, Andrea Burnett, Brian Hall, and Keith K. Parker. Neurochemical Research, Vol. 30, No. 8, August 2005, pp. 1037–1043.

5. *Cannabinoid-related agents in the treatment of anxiety disorders: current knowledge and future perspectives.* Simone Tambaro and Marco Bortolato. Recent Pat CNS Drug Discov. 2012 Apr 1; 7(1): 25–40.

6. *Hypnotic and antiepileptic effects of cannabidiol.* Carlini EA, Cunha JM. J Clin Pharmacol. 1981 Aug-Sep;21(8-9 Suppl):417S-427S.

7. *Opioid Abuse in Chronic Pain — Misconceptions and Mitigation Strategies.* Nora D. Volkow, M.D., and A.

Thomas McLellan, Ph.D. N Engl J Med 2016;
374:1253-1263 March 31, 2016.

8. *Cannabidiol for neurodegenerative disorders: important new clinical applications for this phytocannabinoid?* Fernández-Ruiz J, Sagredo O, Pazos MR, García C, Pertwee R, Mechoulam R, Martínez-Orgado J. Br J Clin Pharmacol. 2013 Feb;75(2):323-33.

9. *Is the cardiovascular system a therapeutic target for cannabidiol?* Stanley CP1, Hind WH, O'Sullivan SE. Br J Clin Pharmacol. 2013 Feb;75(2):313-22.

10. *Cannabidiol lowers incidence of diabetes in non-obese diabetic mice.* Weiss L, Zeira M, Reich S, Har-Noy M, Mechoulam R, Slavin S, Gallily R. Autoimmunity. 2006 Mar;39(2):143-51.

11. The impact of marijuana use on glucose, insulin, and insulin resistance among US adults. Penner EA1, Buettner H, Mittleman MA. Am J Med. 2013 Jul;126(7):583-9.

12. NBC News Reports that Cannabidiol (CBD) "Turns Off" the Cancer Gene Involved in Metastasis Findings. BUSINESSWIRE VIA THE MOTLEY FOOL, AOL.COM. Sep 20th 2012 2:05PM.

13. *Antitumor activity of plant cannabinoids with emphasis on the effect of* cannabidiol *on human breast carcinoma.* Ligresti A, Moriello AS, Starowicz K, Matias I, Pisanti S, De Petrocellis L, Laezza C, Portella G, Bifulco M, Di Marzo V. J Pharmacol Exp Ther. 2006 Sep;318(3):1375-87. Epub 2006 May 25.

14. *Report of a parent survey of cannabidiol-enriched cannabis use in pediatric treatment-resistant epilepsy.* Brenda E. Porter and Catherine Jacobson. Epilepsy Behav. 2013 Dec; 29(3): 574–577.

15. Efficacy and Safety of Epidiolex (Cannabidiol) In Children And Young Adults With Treatment-Resistant Epilepsy: Initial Data From An Expanded Access Program. Orrin Devinsky, Joseph Sullivan, Daniel

Friedman, Elizabeth Thiele, Eric Marsh, Linda Laux, Julie Hedlund, Nicole Tilton, Judith Bluvstein and Maria Cilio. American Epilepsy Society. Annual Meeting Abstracts. 2014.

16. *Cannabidiol enhances anandamide signaling and alleviates psychotic symptoms of schizophrenia.* F M Leweke, D Piomelli, F Pahlisch, D Muhl, C W Gerth, C Hoyer, J Klosterkötter, M Hellmich and D Koethe. Translational Psychiatry 2012.

17. *Cannabidiol exerts sebostatic and antiinflammatory effects on human sebocytes.* Oláh A, Tóth BI, Borbíró I, Sugawara K, Szöllősi AG, Czifra G, Pál B, Ambrus L, Kloepper J, Camera E, Ludovici M, Picardo M, Voets T, Zouboulis CC, Paus R, Bíró T. J Clin Invest. 2014 Sep;124(9):3713-24.

18. *Cannabinoids and glaucoma.* I Tomida,1 R G Pertwee,2 and A Azuara-Blanco. Br J Ophthalmol. 2004 May; 88(5): 708–713.

19. *Medium-Chain Fatty Acids Improve Cognitive Function in Intensively Treated Type 1 Diabetic Patients and Support In Vitro Synaptic Transmission During Acute Hypoglycemia.* Kathleen A. Page, Anne Williamson, Namyi Yu, Ewan C. McNay, James Dzuira, Rory J. McCrimmon, and Robert S. Sherwin. Diabetes. 2009 May; 58(5): 1237–1244.

www.ingramcontent.com/pod-product-compliance
Lightning Source LLC
Chambersburg PA
CBHW060702280326
41933CB00012B/2270